Mitochondria Diet

A 3-Week Plan to Managing Mitochondrial Dysfunction Through Nutrition

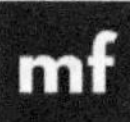

Disclaimer

By reading this disclaimer, you are accepting the terms of the disclaimer in full. If you disagree with this disclaimer, please do not read the guide.

All of the content within this guide is provided for informational and educational purposes only, and should not be accepted as independent medical or other professional advice. The author is not a doctor, physician, nurse, mental health provider, or registered nutritionist/dietician. Therefore, using and reading this guide does not establish any form of a physician-patient relationship.

Always consult with a physician or another qualified health provider with any issues or questions you might have regarding any sort of medical condition. Do not ever dis- regard any qualified professional medical advice or delay seeking that advice because of anything you have read in this guide. The information in this guide is not intended to be any sort of medical advice and should not be used in lieu of any medical advice by a licensed and qualified medical pro- fessional.

The information in this guide has been compiled from a variety of known sources. However, the author cannot attest to or guarantee the accuracy of each source and thus should not be held liable for any errors or omissions.

Table of Contents

Introduction

Did you know that mitochondrial health is an essential key to longevity and overall well-being? Mitochondria, often overlooked in the body's complex cellular structure, play a critical role in maintaining your health.

They may not get as much attention as the brain or heart, but these tiny organelles are integral to overall health. When your cells can't use energy properly from food due to an inability to metabolize glucose, your mitochondrial function suffers. This inefficiency can lead to serious health problems like cardiovascular disease, diabetes, cancer, Alzheimer's Disease, Parkinson's Disease, and more

Fortunately, there are many steps you can take to manage mitochondrial dysfunction through proper nutrition. By focusing on nutrient-dense foods that support mitochondrial health, you can significantly improve your overall well-being.

We have outlined a comprehensive 3-week meal plan designed specifically with your mitochondria in mind, which includes a variety of antioxidant-rich fruits and vegetables, lean proteins, and healthy fats. This plan is intended to provide you with the necessary nutrients to optimize your health and well-being, ensuring that your mitochondria function at their best.

In this guide, you'll discover:

- What mitochondria are
- Diet tips to improve mitochondrial function
- Symptoms indicating your cellular structures aren't working properly
- A seven-day weekly plan
- Sample recipes to follow

Take the first step towards better health by understanding and supporting your mitochondria. Keep reading to learn more about mitochondria and how you can keep them healthy through proper nutrition.

Understanding Mitochondria and Their Function

Mitochondria are often referred to as the powerhouse of the cell. This is because they act as the energy center for your body cells, creating small molecules, such as adenosine triphosphate (ATP), through a process called oxidative phosphorylation.

In other words, they are organelles that help generate energy for cells by converting sugar into usable form and providing essential enzymes to break down fatty acids and amino acids.

Found in most eukaryotic cells, a healthy human adult has thousands, maybe even millions or billions, of mitochondrion—with each playing an essential role in the production of energy. That is, each mitochondrion contains its circular DNA that is separate from the rest of the cell's DNA, which means this type of genetic information is passed down through maternal inheritance only. This allows mitochondrial genetics to be studied in much more detail than nuclear genetics without having to wait for generations of female offspring.

Mitochondria are also responsible for regulating critical genes involved with cellular respiration and signaling pathways, as well as being intimately involved in calcium homeostasis (calcium is an essential nutrient for the cells). Besides their vital role in cellular function, mitochondria can also help prevent disease by regulating inflammation.

In a nutshell, these tiny energy factories work behind the scenes, not only by providing fuel for all cells in our body and creating 90% of our energy supply; they are also vital for our survival. Sometimes though, something goes wrong. There are situations where the mitochondria can get a little too much oxygen, get too few of the required minerals or vitamins, or can't produce enough end products—things the other 98% of the cells in your body can do. Thus, your body has to work harder to get the energy it needs to function. The result can be exhaustion or fatigue, and it can eventually cause other parts of our body to start to malfunction as well.

In other words, when your mitochondria work harder than they should, it increases the likelihood of mitochondrial pathway imbalance, activating their adverse effects.

What Is Mitochondrial Dysfunction or Mitochondrial Disease?

Mitochondrial dysfunction typically is not a disease that has received extensive research, but it can lead to chronic fatigue and other health problems.

It is a term used to refer to any abnormality or impairment in the mitochondria. This dysfunction, or mitophagy, may be caused by genetic mutations or a wide range of factors, like oxidative stress, which happens when the body doesn't have enough antioxidants (natural and/or artificial) to counteract the adverse effects of free radicals.

This condition is also associated with overconsumption of processed foods, heavy metals, and lack of vitamins/minerals, and yes—chances are, if you experience chronic health issues, then this has been the root cause.

Mitochondrial dysfunction is becoming increasingly recognized as a key contributor to several common chronic health problems, including heart disease, multiple sclerosis, diabetes, cancer, and even neurological disorders such as Alzheimer's disease and Parkinson's disease.

Since mitochondrial dysfunction is so often a hidden cause and rarely discussed, most people don't know what's going on, let alone how to treat or manage it. However, you can alter some simple dietary routines to enhance your mitochondrial function. But the first step is to understand what's happening in your body before making these nutritional changes.

Common Types of Mitochondrial Diseases

Mitochondrial diseases are a diverse group of genetic disorders caused by dysfunctional mitochondria, the energy-producing structures within cells.

Here are some of the more common types:

1. **Leber's Hereditary Optic Neuropathy (LHON)**

   Leber's Hereditary Optic Neuropathy (LHON) is a genetic condition that predominantly affects the eyes, leading to sudden and often severe vision loss. This condition typically manifests in young adults, although it can occur at any age.

   The primary impact of LHON is on the optic nerve, which is responsible for transmitting visual information from the eyes to the brain. As the optic nerve degenerates, individuals with LHON experience a rapid decline in their central vision, potentially leading to significant visual impairment or even blindness.

While the peripheral vision may remain unaffected, the loss of central vision can profoundly impact daily activities such as reading, driving, and recognizing faces. LHON is inherited in a mitochondrial pattern, meaning it is passed down from mothers to their children, and it predominantly affects males more than females. Early diagnosis and management are crucial for those affected, as some therapeutic interventions may help slow the progression of the disease.

2. Mitochondrial Myopathy

Mitochondrial Myopathy refers to a group of disorders that significantly impact muscle function due to defects in the mitochondria, which are the energy-producing structures within cells. These disorders lead to a range of symptoms, including muscle weakness, exercise intolerance, and chronic fatigue. Individuals with mitochondrial myopathy may find it difficult to perform physical activities that require sustained effort or endurance, as their muscles are unable to generate adequate energy.

Notable examples of mitochondrial myopathies include Kearns-Sayre Syndrome (KSS) and Progressive External Ophthalmoplegia (PEO). Kearns-Sayre

Syndrome is a rare condition characterized by progressive weakness and paralysis of the eye muscles, leading to drooping eyelids (ptosis) and limited eye movement. It may also involve cardiac conduction defects, hearing loss, and other systemic issues.

On the other hand, Progressive External Ophthalmoplegia primarily affects the muscles controlling eye movement, resulting in similar ocular symptoms, but it can also extend to generalized muscle weakness and involvement of other organ systems.

These disorders are genetically inherited and can vary widely in their severity and presentation. Diagnosis often involves a combination of clinical examination, muscle biopsies, and genetic testing. While there is currently no cure for mitochondrial myopathies, management strategies focus on alleviating symptoms and improving quality of life through supportive care, physical therapy, and targeted treatments to enhance mitochondrial function.

3. Mitochondrial Encephalomyopathy, Lactic Acidosis, and Stroke-like Episodes (MELAS)

Mitochondrial Encephalomyopathy, Lactic Acidosis, and Stroke-like Episodes (MELAS) is a complex and debilitating disorder that can manifest with a wide spectrum of symptoms due to its impact on mitochondrial function. Individuals affected by MELAS often experience muscle weakness, which can range from mild to severe and affect various muscle groups. Seizures are also common in MELAS patients, potentially leading to further neurological complications and requiring careful management.

Recurrent headaches are another hallmark of MELAS, often resembling migraines in their intensity and frequency. These headaches can be debilitating and significantly impact the quality of life. One of the most severe aspects of MELAS is the occurrence of stroke-like episodes, which do not correspond to typical vascular strokes but mimic their symptoms.

These episodes can cause temporary loss of motor skills, such as the ability to walk or move limbs, as well as impairments in speech and vision. The recovery from these episodes can vary, with some individuals regaining abilities over time while others may have lasting deficits.

In addition to these primary symptoms, MELAS can lead to elevated levels of lactic acid in the blood (lactic acidosis), resulting from dysfunctional energy production within the mitochondria. This can cause additional symptoms such as fatigue, muscle pain, and difficulty breathing. The onset of MELAS typically occurs in childhood or early adulthood, but it can present at any age.

4. Myoclonic Epilepsy with Ragged Red Fibers (MERRF)

This disorder is characterized by muscle twitching (myoclonus), generalized epilepsy, and ragged red fibers visible in muscle biopsies. Other symptoms may include hearing loss and short stature. Additional manifestations can involve progressive muscle weakness, exercise intolerance, and sometimes cardiac abnormalities.

MERRF is a mitochondrial disorder, meaning it affects the energy-producing structures within cells. The condition is typically inherited through mutations in mitochondrial DNA, most commonly the MT-TK gene. Regular monitoring and supportive therapies are essential for managing the symptoms and improving the quality of life for those affected.

5. Leigh Syndrome

Leigh Syndrome is a severe neurological disorder that typically arises in infancy or early childhood. It is characterized by progressive loss of mental and movement abilities, which can severely impact the quality of life. Symptoms often include poor sucking ability, loss of head control, and difficulty with feeding.

The condition leads to progressive deterioration of motor skills and cognitive function, often resulting in early death. The disorder is caused by mutations in mitochondrial DNA or nuclear genes affecting mitochondrial function, making it a complex condition to diagnose and treat. Early diagnosis and supportive care can help manage symptoms and improve outcomes temporarily.

6. Neuropathy, Ataxia, and Retinitis Pigmentosa (NARP)

NARP syndrome is a rare genetic disorder that significantly affects the nervous system. It involves sensory neuropathy, which is a type of nerve damage that causes pain, numbness, and tingling sensations often described as "pins and needles." This can be quite debilitating and affect daily activities. People with NARP also experience muscle weakness and ataxia (loss of coordination), making movement difficult and unsteady. This ataxia can lead to frequent falls and difficulty with tasks requiring fine motor skills.

Additionally, NARP causes vision problems due to retinitis pigmentosa, a progressive eye disease that leads to the degeneration of the retina. This results in night blindness and a gradual loss of peripheral vision, eventually leading to tunnel vision. Over time, the vision impairment can become severe, greatly impacting the individual's quality of life. Genetic counseling and supportive therapies are often recommended to manage the symptoms and improve the quality of life for those affected by this challenging syndrome.

Understanding these common types of mitochondrial diseases can help in recognizing symptoms early and seeking appropriate medical care. If you suspect you or a loved one might be affected by a mitochondrial disorder, consulting a healthcare professional specializing in genetics or neurology is crucial for accurate diagnosis and management.

What are the symptoms of mitochondrial dysfunction?

Mitochondrial dysfunction can manifest through a variety of symptoms, which may vary depending on the specific tissues and organs affected. Common symptoms include:

- *Fatigue*: Persistent tiredness and lack of energy are common symptoms since mitochondria are crucial for energy production. This can affect daily activities, making it difficult to maintain normal life routines.
- *Muscle Weakness and Pain*: Muscles may not function properly due to mitochondrial dysfunction, leading to weakness and discomfort. This can manifest as

difficulty in performing physical tasks, muscle cramps, or even chronic pain.

- *Neurological Issues*: Symptoms may include seizures, developmental delays, balance problems, and cognitive difficulties. These neurological issues can significantly impact the quality of life and may require specialized medical care and support.

- *Exercise Intolerance*: Individuals may experience difficulty with physical exertion, often accompanied by prolonged recovery periods after exercise. This can discourage physical activity, further impacting overall health and fitness.

- *Gastrointestinal Problems*: Issues such as bloating, nausea, constipation, or diarrhea may arise due to poor mitochondrial function in the digestive system. These symptoms can disrupt nutritional intake and overall digestion, leading to additional health complications.

- *Cardiovascular Problems*: Heart complications, such as cardiomyopathy or irregular heartbeats, are possible. These cardiovascular issues can be serious and require ongoing medical monitoring and intervention.

- *Respiratory Difficulties*: Shortness of breath or respiratory muscle weakness can occur, making breathing more laborious and less efficient. This may necessitate respiratory therapy or other supportive treatments.

- ***Hearing and Vision Problems***: Loss of hearing or vision may result from nerve damage associated with mitochondrial dysfunction. These sensory impairments can affect communication and daily activities, potentially requiring adaptive devices or therapies.
- ***Poor Growth***: In children, mitochondrial dysfunction can lead to stunted growth and developmental delays. This can impact physical and cognitive development, necessitating a multi-disciplinary approach to care and support.

These symptoms highlight the critical role mitochondria play in various bodily functions and underscore the importance of maintaining mitochondrial health.

Causes of Mitochondrial Dysfunction

Mitochondrial dysfunction can arise from a variety of factors, each of which can significantly impact cellular energy production and overall health.

- ***Genetic Mutations***: Genetic mutations in mitochondrial DNA or nuclear DNA can lead to improper functioning of mitochondrial proteins, affecting the energy production process.
- ***Oxidative Stress***: Excessive free radicals can damage mitochondrial components, impairing their ability to generate ATP efficiently and leading to cellular damage.

- ***Nutrient Deficiencies***: A lack of essential nutrients such as CoQ10, B vitamins, and magnesium can hinder mitochondrial biogenesis and function, reducing energy output.

- ***Environmental Toxins***: Exposure to toxins such as heavy metals, pesticides, and pollutants can disrupt mitochondrial membranes and enzymes, causing dysfunction.

- ***Aging***: As organisms age, the efficiency of mitochondria naturally declines due to accumulated damage from oxidative stress and reduced repair mechanisms.

- ***Infections***: Viral and bacterial infections can negatively impact mitochondrial function either directly through damage or indirectly by inducing inflammatory responses.

- **Inflammation**: Chronic inflammation can lead to mitochondrial dysfunction by altering signaling pathways and increasing oxidative stress within cells.

- ***Poor Lifestyle Choices***: A sedentary lifestyle, unhealthy diet, lack of exercise, and chronic stress can all contribute to impaired mitochondrial function over time.

- ***Medications***: Certain drugs, including some antibiotics and chemotherapeutic agents, may have side effects that disrupt mitochondrial processes.

Addressing these causes is essential for maintaining optimal mitochondrial function and promoting overall health and longevity.

22

Getting to Grips of Mitochondria Dysfunction Through Nutrition

We all know the importance of managing our diet and fitness. However, did you know that it is just as important to manage your mitochondrial health? The mitochondria diet is designed to optimize cellular function through nutrition and lifestyle changes to create a healthier version of ourselves.

This type of diet was recently popularized by Dr. Terry Wahls to reverse chronic disease. According to her, the idea behind the diet is simple: our mitochondria are at the center of every cell in our body, and if they are damaged or deficient in any way, it slows down your metabolism and leads to weight gain and other chronic diseases.

Dr. Wahls further suggests eating foods rich in antioxidants (and thereby anti-inflammatory) such as coenzyme Q10, alpha-lipoic acid, carotenoids, and green tea to protect us against free radicals that damage mitochondria.

Some other tips include avoiding processed food high in fat or sugar because it increases inflammation in the body, harming mitochondria.

Suppose you suspect that your health problems are related to slow-functioning or damaged mitochondria, then it's time to think twice about the mitochondria diet to help you regain your health and boost your mitochondria, too.

Principles of the Mitochondria Diet

The following are the key principles of the mitochondria diet that can help you optimize your cellular function and overall health:

Focus on whole, nutrient-dense foods: Foods that are minimally processed and contain a high amount of nutrients such as vitamins, minerals, antioxidants, and fiber should be the foundation of your diet. These include fruits, vegetables, whole grains, lean proteins, healthy fats, nuts and seeds.

- *Avoid inflammatory foods*: Inflammation is linked to various chronic diseases and can harm mitochondria function. Avoiding highly processed foods, refined sugars and carbohydrates can help reduce inflammation in the body.
- *Incorporate anti-inflammatory herbs and spices*: Adding herbs and spices like turmeric, ginger,

cinnamon, and garlic can help reduce inflammation and support cellular health.

- ***Include healthy fats***: Healthy fats, such as those found in avocados, olive oil, and fatty fish, are essential for mitochondrial function and brain health.
- ***Limit exposure to toxins***: As mentioned earlier, avoiding toxic chemicals is crucial for maintaining optimal mitochondrial function. This includes choosing organic produce whenever possible and using natural cleaning and personal care products.
- ***Stay hydrated***: Drinking enough water is vital for flushing out toxins from the body and supporting cellular processes.
- ***Incorporate intermittent fasting***: Giving your body a break from constant digestion can help improve mitochondrial efficiency and support cellular repair.
- ***Consider supplements***: Adding certain supplements such as CoQ10, magnesium, and B vitamins can help support mitochondrial function and energy production.
- ***Get regular exercise***: Regular exercise not only helps stimulate the growth of new mitochondria but also enhances overall mitochondrial function. Engaging in physical activities such as running, swimming, or weight training can boost your energy levels, improve your metabolism, and contribute to better overall health.
- ***Practice stress management***: Chronic stress can have a negative impact on mitochondrial health. Incorporating

stress-reducing activities such as meditation, yoga or mindfulness practices can be beneficial for both physical and mental well-being.

By adhering to the principles of The Mitochondria Diet, you can optimize your cellular energy production, improve overall well-being, and protect against a range of chronic diseases.

Benefits of the Mitochondria Diet

The Mitochondria Diet offers numerous benefits for both physical and mental health. By supporting cellular function and reducing inflammation, this diet may help:

- ***Increase Energy Levels***: Enhanced mitochondrial function leads to more efficient energy production, resulting in higher overall energy levels.
- ***Improve Cognitive Function***: Better mitochondrial health can support brain function, leading to improved memory, concentration, and mental clarity.
- ***Boost Metabolism***: A healthy diet and active lifestyle can improve metabolic processes, aiding in weight management and reducing the risk of metabolic disorders.
- ***Enhance Exercise Performance***: Optimized energy production and reduced oxidative stress can improve endurance and performance during physical activities.

- ***Support Heart Health***: Nutrient-dense foods and healthy fats support cardiovascular health by reducing inflammation and improving cholesterol levels.
- ***Reduce Inflammation***: Whole, unprocessed foods help lower inflammatory markers, which can alleviate symptoms of chronic diseases and improve overall well-being.
- ***Strengthen Immune System***: A diet rich in antioxidants and essential nutrients supports a robust immune response, helping to ward off infections and illnesses.
- ***Promote Longevity***: By protecting cellular health and reducing the risk of chronic diseases, The Mitochondria Diet can contribute to a longer, healthier life.
- ***Improve Mood and Reduce Stress***: Balanced nutrition and lifestyle practices such as regular exercise and quality sleep can enhance mood and reduce stress levels.
- ***Aid in Disease Prevention***: Supporting mitochondrial function and reducing oxidative stress can help prevent a range of diseases, including diabetes, neurodegenerative disorders, and some types of cancer.

By following the Mitochondria Diet, you can experience these benefits and support your body's natural ability to maintain optimal health and vitality.

Disadvantages of the Mitochondria Diet

While the Mitochondria Diet offers numerous benefits, it's also important to be aware of some potential disadvantages. However, the overall benefits often outweigh these challenges:

1. ***Initial Adjustment Period***: Transitioning to a new diet can be challenging and may require a period of adjustment as your body adapts to healthier food choices and lifestyle changes.

2. ***Time-Consuming Meal Preparation***: Preparing nutrient-dense, whole foods can be time-consuming compared to convenient processed foods. Planning and cooking meals from scratch might take more effort and time.

3. ***Higher Food Costs***: High-quality, organic, and unprocessed foods can be more expensive than processed alternatives. This could increase your food budget.

4. ***Limited Dining Out Options***: Finding suitable options at restaurants and fast-food places might be difficult, limiting your flexibility and convenience when dining out.

5. ***Potential for Nutrient Imbalance***: Without careful planning, there's a risk of missing out on certain nutrients, especially if specific food groups are restricted. It's essential to ensure a balanced intake of all necessary nutrients.

6. ***Requires Consistency and Commitment***: Maintaining the principles of The Mitochondria Diet requires dedication and consistent effort. It can be challenging to stay committed, especially during busy or stressful times.

Despite these disadvantages, the long-term benefits of The Mitochondria Diet—such as improved energy levels, better cognitive function, enhanced overall health, and disease prevention—far outweigh these initial challenges. By committing to this diet, you can significantly enhance your quality of life and well-being.

Nutrients to Include in Your Diet For Mitochondrial Health

Antioxidant-Rich Nutrients

1. ***Coenzyme Q10***, also known as ubiquinone, is a naturally occurring compound that is an integral part of both mitochondrial and cellular energy production. It's often called "the spark of life" because it's an essential part of the process that allows cells to use oxygen and convert food into fuel. It also acts as a natural fat-soluble antioxidant within the body, protecting cells from oxidative damage caused by free radicals.

   Technically, you can find Coenzyme Q10 in some foods like meats, fish, and dairy products; however, it's not always easy to get enough through diet alone. In case you feel like your body is not getting enough of CoQ10 through your dietary sources, you can opt for CoQ10 nutritional supplements to help you protect your cells against oxidative stress and damage.

2. ***Alpha-lipoic acids*** (ALA) is a naturally occurring antioxidant found in many foods like Brussels sprouts, carrots, broccoli, spinach, tomatoes, and potatoes.

   Owing to their antioxidant properties, alpha-lipoic acids can help combat mitochondrial dysfunction by providing additional antioxidants for cells to use during periods when they cannot produce enough on their own due to environmental stress or other factors limiting production.

   It also plays a biogenesis role in the health of mitochondria which includes the formation of new organelles.

3. ***Creatine*** is a naturally synthesized molecule in the liver and the kidneys, primarily found in various types of meat, particularly red meat.

   The influence of creatine on muscle protein synthesis has been studied for its potential to stimulate mitochondrial biogenesis and improve exercise performance. That's because creatine has antioxidant properties that have been shown to stimulate the production of adenosine monophosphate-activated protein kinase (AMPK) and increase the PGC-1 alpha.

AMPK is vital for cellular energy homeostasis and stimulates many pathways that increase cellular metabolism, including mitochondrial biogenesis.

4. ***Carotenoids and Polyphenols Foods.*** Carotenoids are organic pigments that are responsible for the color of many fruits and vegetables. However, phytochemicals found in carotenoids and polyphenols are not only responsible for the color of food, but they also have antioxidative properties associated with neutralizing free radicals before they cause harm to cells or tissues throughout our body.

Therefore, carotenoids and polyphenols can protect mitochondria from damage by inhibiting some of these harmful enzymes. Scientists believe this protection also offers significant health benefits, including slowing down aging processes, preventing cancer and heart disease, decreasing inflammation, improving cognitive function, and boosting immune system defenses.

The best food sources of carotenoids include carrots, sweet potatoes, cantaloupe, apricots, peaches, onions, spinach, kale, tomatoes, collard greens, broccoli, and more.

5. ***Green Tea.*** This contains catechins (flavonoids) that have a free radical scavenging activity and can be used to fight toxins in the body that might pose dangers to your mitochondria.

B Vitamins

The mitochondria are the cell's powerhouse, and their functionality depends on how many nutrients are available to them. Therefore, the welfare of the mitochondria is primarily determined by the number of B vitamins in your system and your body's ability to utilize these vitamins.

The B vitamins are also necessary for the genetic expression of mitochondrial proteins and enzymes involved in energy production. Additionally, B vitamins help maintain the integrity of the mitochondrial membrane by preventing it from becoming too rigid and keeping it fluid and flexible.

Some of the B vitamins to include in your mitochondria diet are:

1. ***Thiamine (vitamin B1)*** is critical in many cellular functions, including ATP production. Therefore, most foods rich in Thiamine are some of our favorite food groups: vegetables, fruits, fish, pork, beef, nuts, legumes, and dried beans.

2. ***Riboflavin (vitamin B2)*** supports the critical mitochondrial enzyme flavin-adenine dinucleotide (FAD), found in the "respiratory chain" used to generate

ATP. Foods rich in vitamin B2 include liver, mushrooms, milk, salmon, yogurt, cheese, and egg yolk.

3. *Niacin (B3)* helps the mitochondria to make energy-producing molecules, which include nicotinamide adenine dinucleotide (NADH) and nicotinamide adenine dinucleotide phosphate (NADPH). These are essential along with ATP, which is produced via glycolysis in supporting the Krebs cycle. As a vitamin, niacin is naturally present in food sources such as fish, lean meats, poultry, fish, whole grains, and legumes.

4. *Pantothenic acid or vitamin B5* is a water-soluble essential nutrient that acts as a coenzyme in multiple metabolic pathways, including beta-oxidation, which is the breakdown of long-chain fatty acids. Pantothenic acid is also known to have anti-inflammatory properties. It can be found abundantly in animal products such as meat, poultry, eggs, milk, and vegetarian sources, including whole grains, legumes, potatoes, nuts, and seeds.

5. *Pyridoxine (vitamin B6)* is one of the less-known vitamins for its role in helping to metabolize protein into energy. It's abundant in liver, fish, eggs, and garbanzo beans. You can also get this B vitamin from wheat germ, oats, bananas, turkey, and potatoes.

6. *Biotin (B7)* functions in the enzymatic reaction. As part of the enzyme propionyl-CoA carboxylase is converted to the branched-chain amino acid valine to propionic

acid in cells such as lymphocytes. Biotin is found in various foods, including nuts, egg yolks, legumes, liver, sunflower seeds, salmon, and sweet potatoes.

7. ***Folate or folic acid (B9)*** functions as a coenzyme in transferring carbon dioxide to under-methylated DNA and RNA precursors, so it is involved in cell reproduction or mitosis. It has also been shown to affect the replication, recombination, and repair of chromosomal DNA. Food sources of B9 include liver, broccoli, black-eyed peas, brussels sprouts, and leafy green vegetables such as kale and spinach.

8. ***Cyanocobalamin (Vitamin B12)*** is a cofactor in a variety of metabolic reactions. As a metabolic cofactor, it assists with the conversion of glucose and fat into energy. Cyanocobalamin also regulates mitochondrial DNA synthesis. Foods rich in Cyanocobalamin include beef, liver, trout, salmon, yogurt, cheese, clams, milk, eggs, and fortified breakfast cereal.

Other Mitochondria Diet Minerals and Vitamins

The mitochondria diet is not just about vitamins, it also includes minerals that are essential for optimal mitochondrial function. Some of these important minerals include:

1. **Zinc**

Zinc acts as a natural antioxidant with anti-inflammatory properties that can help reduce the markers of chronic inflammation caused by oxidative stress by inhibiting free radicals by-products and potentially boosting our mitochondria's longevity.

Loads up on zinc-rich foods such as sprouted legumes, peas, oysters, red meat, cashews, crabs, and fish may help modulate inflammation, supporting mitochondria function.

2. **Magnesium**

Magnesium is an essential mineral that naturally supports mitochondrial energy providers in the body to sustain continuous ATP production (Adenosine Triphosphate), which is the energy molecule utilized by every cell in our body for all metabolic functions, including supporting proper nerve function.

Multiple servings of magnesium-rich foods such as kale, spinach, broccoli, dark chocolate, bananas, whole grains, nuts, pumpkin seeds, almonds, legumes, fatty fish, and avocado will boost the production of beneficial enzymes necessary for mitochondrial function.

3. Iron

Iron is intimately involved in the regulation of the electrons used for ATP generation. Iron-rich foods also help the mitochondria to perform oxidative biochemical reactions where oxygen is a terminal electron acceptor.

Foods high in iron include lentils, apricots, raisins, soybeans, seafood, black-eyed peas, and dark green leafy vegetables. Other good sources of iron are eggs (the yolk is the best source of iron), red meat (especially liver), poultry, and pork. Iron-fortified breakfast cereals are good considerations, too.

4. Sulfur

If you suffer from chronic fatigue and fibromyalgia, you may be interested in foods that are rich in sulfur. The amino acids such as cysteine found in sulfur-rich veggies and prebiotic foods have been shown to prevent aging, promote anti-inflammatory responses, and even stop cellular proliferation, supporting mitochondrial permeability. The most common sulfur-rich foods essential for cellular health are kale, onions, garlic, cruciferous vegetables, chickpeas, cabbage, whole grains, lentils, nuts, and seeds.

5. Vitamin C

This is an essential nutrient found in citrus fruits and other tasty treats such as baked potatoes and kiwi. While it's best known for fighting infections, perhaps its most important function lies in promoting the role of our mitochondria.

Also known as ascorbic acid, it is used in over 100 different metabolic processes in the body and is an important component in collagen production. In our mitochondria, it enables the formation of collagen fibers and maintains cell resistance to oxidative damage by neutralizing free radicals.

6. Vitamin E

This vitamin is an essential dietary supplement to human health that protects the body from free radical damage. Dozens of scientific studies have cropped up, demonstrating that vitamin E has a broad range of benefits—from protecting the brain to boosting longevity.

The specific ingredient that provides these benefits is alpha-tocopherol antioxidants which also play a role in reducing oxidative stress in mitochondria function. If you're looking to restore your mitochondria function, consider including these vitamin E food sources in your diet:

- Sunflower seeds
- Soybean oil
- Paprika

- Almonds
- Peanuts
- Annatto
- Beet greens
- Spinach
- Pumpkin

Avoiding Mitochondria Foods

While your mitochondria use food to generate fuel within the cells, what you eat can be responsible for making your mitochondria healthier or less healthy. Remember, you are only as strong as your mitochondria, meaning that all your moves toward better health will be useless if you have unhealthy mitochondria.

Thus, you should be mindful of the foods you choose to eat since certain food processing may cause degenerative diseases by damaging your mitochondria function.

Here is a list of foods you should avoid in your mitochondria diet:

- Fructose
- Processed foods and meats
- Refined sugars and sweeteners
- Refined grains
- Foods containing gluten
- Alcohol

- Refined carbs
- Foods rich in trans fats

Other Mitochondria Lifestyle Recommendations

Apart from having a healthy diet, other lifestyle changes can improve your mitochondrial health. These include:

Intermittent Fasting

If you don't know, intermittent fasting (IF) is a dietary practice in which you cycle between a period of eating and fasting. One of the most promising aspects of this diet is that it can help you maintain a healthy weight and boost your metabolic and mitochondrial health.

Many people find intermittent fasting to be a more effective form of dieting than traditional calorie restriction. For some, it can be even more effective than low-carb, high-fat diets.

If you want to start intermittent fasting, the easiest way is to skip breakfast. Instead of eating breakfast, you eat something different to satisfy your hunger and avoid overeating. That something could be a smoothie, oatmeal, a smoothie with fruit, almond butter, fruit juice, avocado, peanut butter, almond milk, or any other nutrient-dense food you like.

The key is to find a simple method to hack your mitochondria functions and your central nervous system through biogenesis—the production of newer and healthier organelles.

In addition, when intermittent fasting, the body will burn fat as its primary fuel, increase resistance to stress, regulate hormones, reduce inflammation, and even slow down the aging process, and even help reduce the risk of degenerative diseases.

Exercise

This and your mitochondria are like a match made in health heaven. Exercise improves your body's mitochondrial function by boosting ATP production in your body's cells. Since the body is likely to use more energy, it will develop ways to grow complacent about keeping up with the demand. Another benefit of physical exercise is that it naturally improves your oxygen intake and your mitochondria's Krebs cycle.

Heat Therapy

Heat therapy (or thermal therapy) is commonly used in conventional medicine for chronic musculoskeletal pain, functional disorders, circulation, and injuries. However, mitochondria optimization through the oxidative phosphorylation process resulting from heat therapy is a new concept in the realm of health science to maintain mitochondria efficiency.

You can optimize your mitochondria by having 2-3 heat therapy sessions per week for a minimum of 10-15 minutes in every session.

Detoxification

Our body can naturally detoxify itself in various ways, with the liver and kidneys being the primary organs of detoxification. Still, other systems like the lymphatic system and the nervous system are also involved in the ongoing process of detoxification, which is active every minute of our lives.

Even though detoxification happens every day in our bodies, certain lifestyle choices and external factors can overwhelm our detoxification systems and cause them to become inefficient. Thus, if you're looking for a way to jumpstart your body's ability to detoxify itself, think of it as a cellular cleanse to minimize the toxic load on your mitochondria.

This means avoiding excessive exposure to toxic chemicals that can trigger oxidative stress and cell damage in the mitochondria, triggering a domino effect of health issues and disease.

A 3-Week Mitochondria Diet Plan: How to Do It

Managing your mitochondria health is an ongoing process that involves a combination of various factors, including diet, exercise, and lifestyle choices. However, if you're looking for a specific plan to kickstart your journey to optimizing your mitochondria health, here's a 3-week diet plan that can help.

Mitochondria Diet Plan Week 1

Step 1: Adhere to Clear and Organized Rules and Guidelines

A mitochondria diet is a low-carb, high-fat diet designed to nourish your body and reverse some of the damage caused by your current diet and lifestyle choices. If you have decided to embark on this dietary journey, it's important to note that the first week of the diet is crucial.

This initial week sets the tone for the rest of your journey, laying the foundation for your long-term success. It's a period filled with excitement and nervous energy, but with proper preparation and mindset, you can ensure a smooth transition and a successful start.

To maximize the benefits of the mitochondria diet, it's essential to adhere to simple and structured rules and guidelines. These foundational principles are followed by more flexible steps that you can incorporate as you progress.

The key is to make these changes gradually, as many people experience the most significant benefits from small, incremental adjustments rather than massive overhauls of their lifestyle. Starting with minor changes allows your body to adapt more easily and helps build sustainable habits over time.

During the first week, focus on making manageable adjustments to your eating patterns and daily routines. For example, you might begin by reducing your intake of processed carbohydrates and sugars while increasing your consumption of healthy fats, such as avocados, nuts, and olive oil. Incorporating nutrient-dense, whole foods will provide your body with the necessary fuel to support mitochondrial function and overall well-being.

In addition to dietary changes, consider incorporating other lifestyle modifications that align with the principles of the mitochondria diet. These might include getting adequate sleep, engaging in regular physical activity, and managing stress through mindfulness practices or relaxation techniques. Each of these elements plays a vital role in supporting your body's energy production and cellular health.

Remember, the goal is to create a sustainable and enjoyable approach to your diet and lifestyle. By starting with small, manageable changes, you set yourself up for long-term success and a healthier, more vibrant life. Embrace the journey with patience and persistence, and celebrate each positive step you take along the way.

Step 2: Try the Low-Residue Diet

A low-residue diet is a specialized eating plan that includes foods with minimal fiber content, allowing them to easily pass through the digestive system with reduced effort. This diet is particularly beneficial for individuals who need to manage specific medical conditions or digestive issues, such as Crohn's disease, ulcerative colitis, diverticulitis, or after certain types of surgery. By reducing or eliminating dietary residue—the indigestible parts of food that contribute to stool volume—this diet helps to minimize bowel movements and alleviate symptoms associated with these conditions.

The cornerstone of a low-residue diet is the careful selection of foods that are low in fiber and easy on the digestive tract.

Here are some of the most significant offenders to avoid:

- ***All Fatty Foods***

High-fat foods are difficult to digest and can exacerbate symptoms like bloating, diarrhea, and abdominal discomfort. Examples include fried foods, fatty cuts of meat, and rich sauces. These foods often slow down the digestive process, causing the stomach to work harder and longer, which can lead to increased discomfort and digestive issues over time.

- ***Pastry***

Baked goods made with whole grains, nuts, and seeds are high in fiber and should be avoided. Instead, opt for refined flour products without added fiber. Whole-grain pastries can cause irritation and prolong digestive transit time, which can be problematic for individuals with sensitive digestive systems.

- ***Fruit Juices***

While fruit juices may seem harmless, they often contain pulp or fiber that can irritate the digestive system. Clear fruit juices without pulp are preferable. Even though they might lack fiber, these juices still provide essential vitamins and hydration without causing additional strain on the digestive tract.

- ***Bran Cereals***

Bran is extremely high in fiber. Cereals made with bran or whole grains should be substituted with lower-fiber options such as puffed rice or cornflakes. Bran cereals can be particularly harsh on the digestive system due to their high fiber content, potentially leading to increased bowel movements and discomfort for those needing a low-residue diet.

- ***Corn***

Corn kernels, whether fresh, canned, or in popcorn form, are high in fiber and difficult to digest. It's best to eliminate them from your diet while following a low-residue plan. Corn's fibrous outer shell can be tough on the digestive tract and often leads to bloating and other gastrointestinal discomforts, making it unsuitable for those needing to minimize their fiber intake.

In addition to avoiding these high-residue foods, it is crucial to focus on what you can eat. Foods recommended on a low-residue diet often include:

- ***Refined Grains***

White bread, plain bagels, white rice, and pasta made from refined flour are all low in fiber and easier on the digestive system. These grains have been processed to remove the bran and germ, resulting in a finer texture and longer shelf life but less nutritional value compared to whole grains.

- ***Lean Proteins***

Skinless poultry, fish, eggs, and tofu provide necessary protein without adding excessive residue. These proteins are essential for muscle repair and growth while being easier to digest compared to fatty cuts of meat.

- ***Cooked Vegetables***

Well-cooked, peeled vegetables like carrots, green beans, and potatoes (without skins) are more digestible and less likely to irritate. Cooking vegetables breaks down some of the fiber, making them gentler on the digestive tract while still offering essential vitamins and minerals.

- ***Dairy***

Milk, yogurt, and cheese can be included in moderation, provided you do not have lactose intolerance. Dairy products are excellent sources of calcium and vitamin D, which are important for bone health, but should be consumed carefully to avoid digestive discomfort.

- ***Clear Soups and Broths***

These are gentle on the stomach and help maintain hydration. Clear soups and broths can provide electrolytes and nutrients in a form that is easily digestible, making them great options for those with sensitive stomachs or during recovery from illness.

Transitioning to a low-residue diet involves careful planning and a focus on food preparation techniques that reduce fiber content, such as peeling and thoroughly cooking vegetables. As with any dietary plan tailored for medical conditions, it is essential to consult with a healthcare provider before making significant changes to ensure that the diet meets your nutritional needs while managing your symptoms effectively.

Step 3: Replace High-Glycemic Foods

High-glycemic foods, also known as high-glycemic-index (GI) foods, are rapidly absorbed into the bloodstream, causing a swift and significant rise in blood glucose levels. This rapid spike in blood sugar can lead to increased inflammation—a key factor in mitochondrial dysfunction and various chronic health conditions. High-glycemic foods typically include refined grains, sugary snacks, and processed carbohydrates, which can wreak havoc on your metabolic health when consumed in excess.

To mitigate these effects, a crucial step in optimizing your diet is to trim down your grain intake and replace high-glycemic foods with low-glycemic alternatives. By doing so, you can achieve better blood sugar stability and reduce the risk of excessive fat accumulation. Here's a more detailed look at how to make these changes effectively:

Understanding High-Glycemic Foods

High-glycemic foods are characterized by their ability to cause rapid increases in blood sugar. Common examples include:

- **White Bread and Pastries**: These refined grain products are stripped of fiber and essential nutrients during processing, leading to quick glucose absorption and rapid spikes in blood sugar levels. Consistent consumption can contribute to health issues like diabetes and obesity.

- **Sugary Cereals and Snacks**: Items such as candy, sweetened breakfast cereals, and baked goods loaded with sugar are notorious for spiking blood sugar levels. These foods provide a quick energy boost but can lead to crashes, making it difficult to maintain a balanced energy level throughout the day.

- **White Rice and Pasta**: Though staples in many diets, these refined carbohydrates can cause significant blood sugar surges due to their low fiber content. Incorporating whole grains as an alternative can help in maintaining more stable blood sugar levels and provide additional health benefits.

Embracing Low-Glycemic Foods

Low-glycemic foods are digested and absorbed more slowly, resulting in gradual increases in blood sugar and providing longer-lasting energy. These foods are rich in nutrients and fiber, making them excellent substitutes for high-glycemic options.

Some examples include:

- **Non-Starchy Vegetables**: Vegetables like leafy greens, broccoli, cauliflower, zucchini, and bell peppers are low in carbohydrates and high in fiber, vitamins, and minerals.
- **Fruits**: While fruits contain natural sugars, many have a low glycemic index. Berries, apples, pears, and citrus fruits are great choices that provide essential nutrients without drastically affecting blood sugar levels.
- **Whole Grains**: Opt for whole grains like quinoa, barley, and oats, which are higher in fiber and take longer to digest, resulting in more stable blood glucose levels.
- **Legumes**: Beans, lentils, and chickpeas are excellent sources of both protein and low-glycemic carbohydrates, contributing to sustained energy release.
- **Nuts and Seeds**: Almonds, walnuts, chia seeds, and flaxseeds offer healthy fats, protein, and fiber, helping to keep blood sugar levels in check.

Practical Tips for Transitioning

1. Meal Planning

Start by planning your meals around low-glycemic foods to help stabilize blood sugar levels. Incorporate a variety of colorful vegetables, such as leafy greens, bell peppers, and carrots, as well as lean proteins like chicken, fish, and legumes. Don't forget to include healthy fats from sources like avocados, nuts, and olive oil to create balanced, nutritious meals.

2. *Read Labels*

Be mindful of food labels and ingredients. Take the time to check for hidden sugars, artificial additives, and unhealthy fats. Avoid products with added sugars and refined carbohydrates, as they can contribute to health issues like weight gain and diabetes. Instead, opt for natural, whole foods with minimal processing to ensure you're making healthier choices.

3. *Cooking Methods*

Choose cooking methods that preserve the nutritional integrity of low-glycemic foods. Steaming, roasting, and grilling are preferable to frying or overly-processing foods, as these methods help retain essential vitamins and minerals. Additionally, these techniques can enhance the natural flavors of the ingredients, making your meals both healthier and more delicious.

4. *Mindful Eating*

Practice mindful eating by chewing slowly and savoring each bite. Take the time to appreciate the flavors, textures, and aromas of your food. This not only aids digestion but also helps you tune into your body's hunger and satiety signals, allowing you to make more conscious and healthier eating choices.

By prioritizing low-glycemic foods, you support better blood sugar management, reduce inflammation, and promote overall mitochondrial health. Making these dietary adjustments can be a powerful step towards achieving a balanced, nutrient-rich diet that enhances your well-being.

Step 4: Stay Hydrated

Water is essential for life. Our bodies depend on adequate hydration to function optimally, as every cell, tissue, and organ requires water to operate efficiently. Proper hydration plays a crucial role in maintaining overall health by facilitating various physiological processes, including toxin elimination, nutrient transport, temperature regulation, and joint lubrication.

Importance of Hydration

Water is fundamental to our biological functions. Here are some key ways in which staying hydrated supports your well-being:

- *Cellular Function*: Water is vital for cellular hydration, allowing cells to maintain their shape, structure, and function effectively. Proper hydration supports various cellular processes, including nutrient transport and waste removal. It also plays a crucial role in the production of energy within cells, ensuring they function optimally.

- ***Detoxification***: Adequate water intake helps the kidneys efficiently flush out toxins and waste products from the bloodstream, promoting a clean and healthy internal environment. By supporting kidney function, water aids in reducing the risk of kidney stones and urinary tract infections.

- ***Digestion and Nutrient Absorption***: Water is essential for breaking down food, ensuring that nutrients are absorbed efficiently in the digestive tract. It helps form saliva and digestive juices, facilitating smoother digestion and preventing constipation by maintaining stool consistency.

- ***Joint Health***: Water acts as a lubricant for joints, reducing friction and preventing discomfort during movement. Proper hydration supports the production of synovial fluid, which cushions and protects joints, reducing the likelihood of joint pain and stiffness.

- ***Temperature Regulation***: Through processes like sweating and respiration, water helps regulate body temperature, keeping it within a safe range. By dissipating heat through sweat, water prevents overheating and supports the body's ability to function in various environmental conditions.

How Much Water Do You Need?

While individual hydration needs can vary based on factors such as age, weight, activity level, and climate, a general guideline is to increase your fluid intake to at least 3 liters per day. This amount helps ensure that your body remains well-hydrated and can perform its essential functions effectively.

Practical Tips for Staying Hydrated

To maintain optimal hydration levels, consider incorporating these practical tips into your daily routine:

- ***Consistent Water Intake***: Spread your water consumption throughout the day rather than drinking large amounts at once. Aim to drink a glass of water with each meal and snack. This helps ensure that your body is consistently hydrated without overwhelming your system at any one time.
- ***Carry a Water Bottle***: Keep a reusable water bottle with you at all times as a reminder to drink water regularly. Opt for a bottle with measurement markers to track your intake. Having a water bottle within arm's reach makes it easier to take frequent sips and maintain good hydration habits.
- ***Infused Water***: If plain water feels monotonous, infuse it with natural flavors by adding slices of lemon, cucumber, mint, or berries. This can make hydration more enjoyable by adding a refreshing twist to your drink, which might encourage you to drink more water throughout the day.

- ***Monitor Urine Color***: A simple way to gauge your hydration status is by checking the color of your urine. Light yellow or clear urine typically indicates good hydration, while darker urine suggests the need for more fluids. This method is a quick and effective way to ensure you are meeting your body's hydration needs.

- ***Hydrate Before, During, and After Exercise***: Physical activity increases your body's need for water. Drink water before starting your workout to prepare your body, take regular sips during exercise to maintain hydration levels, and ensure you rehydrate afterward to replace the fluids lost through sweat.

- ***Eat Water-Rich Foods***: Incorporate foods with high water content into your diet. Fruits like watermelon, oranges, and strawberries, as well as vegetables like cucumber, lettuce, and celery, contribute to your overall hydration. These foods not only help keep you hydrated but also provide essential vitamins and nutrients that support overall health.

Benefits of Staying Well-Hydrated

Maintaining adequate hydration offers numerous benefits beyond basic physiological functions:

- ***Improved Cognitive Function***: Staying hydrated supports brain function by ensuring that your brain cells receive the necessary oxygen and nutrients, which enhances concentration, memory, and mood. Adequate hydration can also help prevent headaches and improve mental clarity.

- ***Enhanced Physical Performance***: Proper hydration helps maintain muscle function and endurance by keeping your muscles well-lubricated and nourished. This reduces the risk of cramps and fatigue during physical activities, allowing you to perform at your best for longer periods.

- ***Healthy Skin***: Water helps keep your skin hydrated, promoting elasticity and a healthy complexion. Adequate hydration can also help flush out toxins from your skin, reducing the risk of acne and giving your skin a natural glow.

- ***Weight Management***: Drinking water before meals can aid in appetite control by making you feel full sooner, which helps prevent overeating. Additionally, water can support your metabolism and assist in the breakdown of fats, making it a valuable component of any weight management efforts.

By making a conscious effort to stay well-hydrated, you empower your body to function at its best, supporting overall health and vitality. Remember, water is not just a necessity; it is a cornerstone of a healthy lifestyle.

Mitochondria Diet Plan Week 2

In week 2 of the Mitochondria Diet Plan, we will focus on building upon the foundations laid in week 1. This week, we will incorporate more nutrient-dense foods that are rich in antioxidants and essential vitamins and minerals to further support mitochondrial function.

Step 5: Start a food plan

As discussed above, the Mitochondria Diet involves nutrients known to support metabolism and stable mitochondrial function by minimizing the odds of inflammation and blood glucose levels.

The food plan dietary category involves the three types of macronutrients (carbohydrates, proteins, and fats), which offer calories for nutrients. In a nutshell, this food plan is designed as a bold print of the suggested foods to choose from each day in each category. These food items are:

1. *Proteins*
   - Salmon
   - Fish
   - Shrimp
   - Beef
   - Chicken
   - Turkey
   - Egg
   - Mushroom

- Whey Protein

2. *Dairy Alternatives (Proteins + Carbs)*
    - Buttermilk
    - Coconut milk
    - Cashew Milk
    - Hemp milk
    - Yogurt

3. *Fats & Oil*
    - Avocado oil
    - Extra virgin olive oil
    - Coconut ghee
    - Avocado
    - Coconut milk
    - Grapeseed oil
    - Sunflower
    - Walnut
    - Pumpkin
    - Butter
    - Dark chocolate

4. *Starchy Vegetables (Carbs)*
    - Acorn squash
    - Beets
    - Butternut Squash
    - Parsnip
    - Potatoes
    - Chicken peas

5. _Non-Starchy Vegetables (Carbs)_
   - Arugula
   - Turnips
   - Mushrooms
   - Persley
   - Lettuce
   - Kale
   - Salsa
   - Tomatoes
   - Chestnuts
   - Squash
   - Leeks
   - Zucchini
   - Fennel
   - Carrots
   - Cucumbers
   - Sprouts
   - Okra
   - Spinach
   - Asparagus
   - Broccoli
   - Cauliflower
   - Brussels sprouts
   - Cabbage
   - Shallots

6. _Fruits_
   - Blackberries

- Lemon
- Lime
- Avocado
- Apple
- Blueberries
- Cherries
- Grapes
- Mango
- Raspberries
- Strawberries
- Apricots, fresh
- Banana
- Kiwi
- Orange
- Papaya
- Peach

7. *Legumes (Protein + Carbs)*
    - Lentils
    - Beans
    - Peas

8. *Nut & Seeds (Protein + Carbs)*
    - Hemp Seeds
    - Almond
    - Chia seeds
    - Flaxseeds
    - Pumpkin seeds
    - Cashews

- Peanuts
- Sesame seeds
- Pine nuts
- Soy nuts
- Sunflower seeds toasted

9. *Gluten-free carbs*
   - Oats
   - Corn
   - Brown-rice
   - Quinoa

10. *Spices*
   - Rosemary needles
   - Black pepper
   - Sea salt
   - Garlic
   - Thyme leaves
   - Onions
   - Red pepper
   - Cumin
   - Paprika
   - Kosher salt

Mitochondria Diet Week 3

Weekly Diet Plan: A 7-day sample meal plan to follow

Here is a sample meal plan made for a week that you can either follow or modify accordingly. The purpose of creating a meal plan is to help you watch what you are about to consume and make sure you're meeting your daily nutrition needs.

Sample Recipes

We have included a few sample recipes for you to try out while following this meal plan. These recipes are not only delicious but also nutritious and packed with ingredients that support mitochondrial health.

Avocado and Quinoa Salad

Ingredients:

- 4 avocados cut into pieces
- 1 cup of quinoa
- 400 grams of chickpeas
- 30 grams of fresh parsley

Instructions:

1. Rinse the quinoa in a strainer until the water runs clear.
2. In a medium saucepan, add 1 cup of quinoa and 2 cups of water. Bring to a boil, reduce heat, and simmer for 15 minutes or until the water is absorbed.
3. Remove from heat, fluff with a fork, and let cool.
4. In a separate bowl, mix together avocados, chickpeas, and fresh parsley.
5. Add cooked quinoa to the mixture and toss gently.
6. Serve cold as a salad or use it as a side dish for your main meal.

Baked Spinach and Cheese Omelets

Ingredients:

- 10 large eggs
- 1/2 cup of milk or milk alternative
- Salt and pepper to taste
- 200 grams of spinach, chopped
- 200 grams of shredded cheese (cheddar or mozzarella work well)

Instructions:

1. Preheat your oven to 375°F (190°C).
2. In a mixing bowl, beat the eggs with milk, salt, and pepper.
3. Add in the chopped spinach and mix well.
4. Pour the mixture into a greased baking dish.
5. Sprinkle shredded cheese on top evenly.
6. Bake for 30 minutes or until the edges are golden and the middle is set.
7. Let it cool for a few minutes before slicing into squares or wedges.
8. Serve warm as a breakfast meal or save leftovers for a quick and nutritious snack.

Turkey Avocado Wrap

Ingredients:

- 4 whole grain tortillas
- 1 avocado, mashed
- 8 slices of deli turkey meat
- Handful of baby spinach leaves

Instructions:

1. Lay out the tortillas on a flat surface.
2. Divide the mashed avocado evenly between the tortillas and spread it over each one.
3. Place two slices of deli turkey meat on top of the avocado.
4. Add a handful of baby spinach leaves on top of the turkey slices.
5. Roll up the wraps tightly.
6. Cut in half or slice into bite-sized pieces for a party snack.
7. Serve immediately or store in the fridge for later.

Chicken Coconut Milk Soup

Ingredients:

- 1 tablespoon of coconut oil
- 1 onion, diced
- 3 cloves of garlic, minced
- 2 chicken breasts, diced
- 1 can of coconut milk
- 4 cups of chicken broth
- Juice of one lime
- Salt and pepper to taste

Instructions:

1. Heat up a large pot over medium heat.
2. Add in the coconut oil and let it melt.
3. Sauté the onions and garlic until fragrant.
4. Add in the diced chicken breast and cook until no longer pink.
5. Pour in the coconut milk and chicken broth.
6. Let the soup simmer for 10-15 minutes.
7. Add in the lime juice, salt, and pepper to taste.
8. Serve hot and enjoy the creamy and flavorful soup.

Beef Butternut Squash Vegetables Stew

Ingredients:

- 1 tablespoon of olive oil
- 1 onion, chopped
- 2 cloves of garlic, minced
- 1 pound of beef stew meat, cut into cubes
- 2 cups of cubed butternut squash
- 1 can of diced tomatoes
- 2 cups of beef broth
- Salt and pepper to taste

Instructions:

1. Heat the olive oil in a large pot over medium heat.
2. Sauté the onions and garlic until fragrant.
3. Add in the beef stew meat and cook until browned.
4. Pour in the beef broth and bring to a boil.
5. Reduce heat to a simmer and add in the cubed butternut squash.
6. Let the stew cook for 20-25 minutes, until the beef is tender.
7. Stir in the can of diced tomatoes and let it simmer for an additional 10 minutes.
8. Season with salt and pepper to taste.
9. Serve hot and enjoy this hearty and nutritious stew.

Roasted Veggies

Ingredients:

- 1/2 lb. turnips
- 1/2 lb. carrots
- 1/2 lb. parsnips
- 2 shallots, peeled
- 1/4 tsp. ground black pepper
- 1 tbsps. extra-virgin olive oil
- 6 cloves garlic
- 3/4 tsp. kosher salt
- 2 tbsp. fresh rosemary needles

Instructions:

1. First, cut vegetables into bite-sized pieces.
2. Set the oven to 400°F.
3. Mix all the ingredients in a baking dish.
4. Roast the vegetables for 25 minutes until brown and tender.
5. Toss and roast again for 20- 25 minutes.
6. Serve and enjoy while hot.

Zucchini and Celery Greens Soup

Ingredients:

- 1/2 cup cooked green lentils
- 1 onion, finely diced
- 1 parsnip, peeled and finely diced
- 2 garlic cloves, crushed
- 1 green bell pepper, cut into small cubes
- 1 zucchini, sliced
- 4 asparagus spears
- 1 fennel bulb, diced finely
- 2 celery stalks, diced finely
- 1 small bunch of celery greens or other greens available: beet greens, kale, or spinach

- 2 cups low-sodium vegetable broth
- 1 lime, juice only
- 1 tsp. Chia seeds to garnish
- freshly ground black pepper

Instructions:

1. In a large pot, add water and bring it to a boil.
2. Add onions, garlic, parsnip, bell pepper, zucchini, asparagus spears, fennel bulb, and celery stalks.
3. Cook for 10 minutes until vegetables are soft.
4. Pour in the vegetable broth and let it simmer for 5-7 minutes.

5. Add cooked green lentils and greens of your choice.

6. Simmer for another 5 minutes until all the flavors blend together.

7. Squeeze in lime juice and stir well.

8. Serve hot with chia seeds and freshly ground black pepper on top for added texture and flavor.

Salmon Soup

Ingredients:

- 1-3/4 cup coconut milk
- 2 tsp. dried thyme leaves
- 4 gluten-free leeks, trimmed and sliced into crescents
- 6 cups seafood stock or chicken broth
- salt, for seasoning
- 3 cloves garlic, minced
- 1 lb. salmon, cut into bite-sized pieces
- 2 tbsp. avocado oil

Instructions:

1. In a large pot, heat avocado oil over medium heat.
2. Add leeks and garlic, and sauté until fragrant and soft.
3. Pour in seafood stock or chicken broth, and let it simmer for 10 minutes.
4. Stir in coconut milk and dried thyme leaves.
5. Season with salt according to your taste preference.
6. Carefully add salmon pieces into the soup and cook for another 5-7 minutes until fully cooked.
7. Serve hot with your favorite gluten-free bread or crackers on the side. Enjoy!

Baked Bean Vegetables Soup

Ingredients:

- 1 can of organic baked beans
- 2 cups low-sodium vegetable broth
- 3 medium-sized carrots, peeled and diced
- 2 celery stalks, chopped
- 1 medium-sized onion, diced
- 1 red bell pepper, seeded and diced
- 1 cup diced tomatoes

Instructions:

1. Preheat oven to 375°F (190°C).
2. In a large pot or Dutch oven, mix together baked beans, vegetable broth, carrots, celery, onion, red bell pepper, and tomatoes.
3. Cover the pot and place it in the oven for 30-40 minutes, stirring occasionally.
4. Once vegetables are tender, remove them from heat and let them cool for a few minutes.
5. Use an immersion blender to puree the soup until smooth or transfer it to a blender and blend until desired consistency is reached.
6. Serve hot with crusty bread on the side. Enjoy!

Seafood Stew

Ingredients:

- 2 tsp. extra-virgin olive oil
- 1 cut bulb fennel
- 2 stalks celery, chopped
- 2 cups white wine
- 1 tbsp. chopped thyme
- 1 cup chopped shallots
- 6 ounces shrimp
- 6 ounces of sea scallops
- 1/4 tsp. salt
- 1 cup chopped parsley
- 6 oz. Arctic char
- 2-1/2 cups of water

Instructions:

1. In a large saucepan, heat olive oil over medium heat.
2. Add chopped fennel and celery, and cook until tender.
3. Pour in white wine and let it simmer for 5 minutes.
4. Stir in thyme, shallots, shrimp, sea scallops, salt, and parsley into the mixture.
5. Cook for another 5-7 minutes until seafood is fully cooked.

6. Gently place Arctic char on top of the stew.

7. Reduce heat to low and cover the pan with a lid for 10 minutes or until the fish flakes easily with a fork.

8. Serve hot and enjoy this delicious seafood stew with a side of crusty bread or rice.

Tahini Salmon

Instructions:

- 1/4 cup tahini
- 3 tbsp. fresh lemon juice
- 1 tsp. mashed garlic
- 1/4 tsp. salt
- 1/2 cup finely chopped cilantro
- 2 tbsp. roughly chopped toasted walnuts
- 2 tbsp. roughly chopped toasted almonds
- 1 tbsp. finely chopped onion
- 1 tsp. extra-virgin olive oil
- cayenne (gluten-free)
- black pepper, freshly ground
- 1 lb. wild salmon skin removed, fresh or frozen

Instructions:

1. In a mixing bowl, combine tahini, lemon juice, garlic and salt.
2. Whisk the mixture until it becomes smooth.
3. Add cilantro, walnuts, almonds, onion, and olive oil to the bowl and mix well.
4. Preheat your oven to 375°F (190°C).
5. Season both sides of the salmon with cayenne and black pepper.
6. Place the salmon in a baking dish lined with parchment paper.

7. Spread the tahini mixture evenly over the top of the salmon fillet.

8. Bake for 15-20 minutes or until the fish is cooked through.

9. Serve with a side of roasted vegetables or quinoa for a complete meal.

Vegetable Broth

Ingredients:

- 1 tbsp. oil
- 2 leeks, sliced
- 2 carrots, sliced
- 2 ribs celery
- 1/4 tsp. salt
- 8 cups water

To make the soup:

- 1 tbsp. oil
- 2 cups potatoes, diced
- 1 cup mushrooms, diced
- 1-1/2 cups cauliflower, diced
- 1 cup onion, diced
- 1 cup celery, diced
- 1 cup carrot, diced
- 1-1/2 cups red beans, cooked
- 2 sprigs rosemary
- 4 sprigs thyme
- 2 cups spinach

Instructions:

1. To a pot on medium heat, add oil and leeks.
2. Cook for about three minutes or until they start to soften up.

3. Add carrots and top a few celery stalks with leaves.

4. Cover with water.

5. Add salt. Bring to a simmer and cook until carrots are very tender but not mushy.

6. Turn off the heat and let it cool down a little.

7. When the broth has cooled down, strain out the veggies.

8. Remove carrots and set them aside.

9. Squeeze most of the liquid out of the leeks and celery.

To cook the soup:

1. Add carrots to some of the broth and blend.

2. With a pot on medium heat, add oil, onions, raw carrots, and celery. Cook until onions are translucent, approximately 3 to 5 minutes.

3. Add broth, potatoes, and herbs.

4. Bring to a simmer and cook for 10 minutes.

5. Add cauliflower and red beans.

6. Simmer for another 5 minutes.

7. Add the package of frozen green beans and cook until the potatoes and cauliflower are tender, approximately for another 5 minutes.

8. At the end of cooking, add spinach.

9. Serve warm.

Mixed Bone Broth

Ingredients:

- 2 lbs. mixed beef bones, neck bones, oxtails, short ribs, and knuckles
- 2 tbsp. Apple cider vinegar
- water
- 1 large carrot
- 1 large yellow onion

Instructions:

1. Preheat the oven to 400°F.
2. Set up a rack in the middle of the oven. Leave it to preheat to 400°F.
3. Run cold water over the bones and pat dry with paper towels.
4. Put the bones on a rimmed baking sheet. Roast in the oven until golden brown.
5. Transfer the bones to a large stockpot or slow cooker. Add water until it covers everything.
6. Add the vinegar and stir well. Place the lid on and allow the pot to sit for 30 minutes.
7. Bring the pot to a simmer over high heat.
8. Skim the broth for the first hour, then immediately turn down the heat to the lowest setting.
9. Skim off the foam on the surface. Add water as needed to keep the water level. Cover the pan.

10. Set to simmer on low for 24 hours.

11. Add carrots and onions and cook for another 12 to 24 hours.

12. If the broth has a rich golden-brown color and the bones are separating from the joints, it's already done.

13. Strain the broth to separate the solids at once. Discard the bones and vegetables.

14. Fill a basin with cold water and ice. It should be big enough to hold the pot or container where the broth is. Place the pot in the ice bath.

15. Stir until the broth is about 50°F

16. Transfer to airtight jars or containers before freezing or putting them in the fridge.

Pine Nut Quinoa Bowl

Ingredients:

- 1 cup quinoa
- 2 cups water or broth of choice
- 1 tbsp. olive oil
- 1 onion, chopped
- 2 cloves garlic, minced
- 1 red bell pepper, diced
- ½ cup pine nuts

Instructions:

1. Rinse the quinoa in a fine mesh strainer and drain well.
2. In a medium saucepan, bring the water or broth to a boil over high heat.
3. Add the quinoa and reduce the heat to low. Cover and simmer for about 15 minutes until all the water is absorbed.
4. Meanwhile, heat olive oil in a medium skillet over medium-high heat.
5. Add onions and cook until they begin to soften about 3 minutes.
6. Add garlic and red bell pepper and cook for an additional 2 minutes.
7. Stir in pine nuts and continue cooking until vegetables are tender and pine nuts are lightly toasted.

8. Fluff the cooked quinoa with a fork and transfer it to a
    serving bowl.
9. Top with the sautéed vegetables and pine nuts.
10. Serve hot or cold as desired.

Conclusion

Thank you for taking the time to delve into our guide on Mitochondria Disease and the Mitochondria Diet. By diving into this comprehensive resource, you have taken a crucial step toward understanding not only the complexities of mitochondrial disease but also how diet plays a vital role in managing it. Your commitment to learning and improving your health is truly commendable.

Living with mitochondrial disease can present many challenges, but it's important to remember that knowledge is a powerful tool. By educating yourself about the condition and how to support your health through a mitochondria-friendly diet, you are equipping yourself with the means to make positive changes. Every piece of information you've absorbed here can be a stepping stone toward better health and well-being.

Embracing a mitochondrial diet is not merely about following dietary recommendations—it's about adopting a lifestyle that aligns with your body's needs. Foods rich in antioxidants, healthy fats, and essential nutrients play a significant role in supporting your mitochondria. These nutrients help combat oxidative stress, provide the building blocks for cellular energy, and support overall bodily functions. By selecting these foods, you are actively contributing to the health and efficiency of your mitochondria.

Remember, hydration, exercise, and proper sleep are as critical as the food you consume. Staying hydrated ensures that your cells function optimally, regular exercise stimulates the creation of new mitochondria, and adequate sleep allows your body to repair and rejuvenate. Incorporating these elements into your daily routine can make a substantial difference in how you feel and function.

While making dietary and lifestyle changes can be beneficial, don't hesitate to seek professional guidance. Nutritionists and healthcare providers with expertise in mitochondrial diseases can offer personalized advice tailored to your specific needs. They can help you navigate your diet and lifestyle adjustments, ensuring that you receive the most effective care possible.

Being proactive about your health is empowering. It allows you to take control and make informed decisions that positively impact your well-being. Progress may come in small steps, but each one is worth celebrating. Every healthy choice you make is a victory that contributes to your overall health and resilience.

Support networks are invaluable on this journey. Connecting with others who understand your experiences can provide emotional support and practical tips. Whether through online communities, local support groups, or friends and family, having a network of supportive individuals can make a significant difference.

Continuing to educate yourself about mitochondrial health is also crucial. Stay updated with the latest research and advancements. Science is always evolving, and new discoveries can offer additional strategies for managing mitochondrial diseases more effectively. By staying informed, you can adapt and refine your approach as new information becomes available.

As you move forward, remember that living with mitochondrial disease and following a mitochondria-friendly diet are journeys, not destinations. It's okay to take things one step at a time and to be kind to yourself along the way. Each positive decision you make brings you closer to a healthier, more vibrant life.

Your dedication to understanding and managing mitochondrial disease through informed dietary choices and lifestyle changes are truly inspiring. Thank you again for investing your time in this guide. Your journey toward optimized mitochondrial health is a remarkable one, and we are honored to be part of it. Keep pushing forward with courage and confidence, knowing that every step you take is a step towards a brighter, healthier future.

Frequently Asked Questions (FAQs)

What is mitochondrial disease?

Mitochondrial disease refers to a group of disorders caused by dysfunctional mitochondria, the energy-producing structures within cells. These diseases can affect various parts of the body, often leading to symptoms like muscle weakness, fatigue, neurological issues, and organ dysfunction.

How is mitochondrial disease diagnosed?

Diagnosing mitochondrial disease can be complex and typically involves a combination of clinical evaluations, genetic testing, imaging studies, and sometimes muscle biopsies. A specialist, such as a neurologist or geneticist, often coordinates these tests to confirm a diagnosis.

Can diet impact mitochondrial disease?

Yes, diet can significantly impact mitochondrial disease. Certain nutrients support mitochondrial function and help manage symptoms. A diet rich in antioxidants, healthy fats, vitamins, and minerals can help reduce oxidative stress and enhance cellular energy production, thereby supporting overall mitochondrial health.

What foods are beneficial for mitochondrial health?

Foods that are beneficial for mitochondrial health include those rich in antioxidants (such as berries, leafy greens, and nuts), healthy fats (like avocados, olive oil, and fatty fish), and essential nutrients (including whole grains, lean proteins, and legumes). These foods help protect mitochondria from damage and support their function.

Are there specific supplements recommended for mitochondrial disease?

Certain supplements may be recommended for individuals with mitochondrial disease, including Coenzyme Q10 (CoQ10), L-carnitine, and various vitamins (such as B vitamins and vitamin E). However, it's important to consult with a healthcare provider before starting any new supplements, as they can tailor recommendations to your specific needs.

How does exercise affect mitochondrial function?

Regular exercise can positively impact mitochondrial function by stimulating the production of new mitochondria and enhancing their efficiency. Activities like aerobic exercise, strength training, and flexibility exercises can help improve overall mitochondrial health and energy levels.

Can lifestyle changes improve symptoms of mitochondrial disease?

Yes, lifestyle changes can help improve symptoms of mitochondrial disease. Besides following a mitochondria-friendly diet, staying hydrated, getting regular exercise, managing stress, and ensuring adequate sleep are all critical components of a holistic approach to managing mitochondrial disease and improving overall quality of life. Consulting with healthcare professionals for personalized guidance is also crucial.

References and Helpful Links

Meals, M. (2023, December 18). 10 ways to boost your mitochondria. Metabolic Meals - Blog. https://blog.mymetabolicmeals.com/mitochondria-health/

Dminich, & Dminich. (2023, December 15). What to eat to fuel a healthy mitochondria | Deanna Minich. Deanna Minich. https://deannaminich.com/what-to-eat-to-fuel-a-healthy-mitochondria/

Jornayvaz, F. R., & Shulman, G. I. (2010). Regulation of mitochondrial biogenesis. Essays in Biochemistry, 47, 69–84. https://doi.org/10.1042/bse0470069

The Institute for Functional Medicine. (2024, July 9). Therapeutic food plans: a component of personalized nutrition. https://www.ifm.org/news-insights/new-online-learning-course-developed-ifm-ana/

Newman, T. (2023, June 14). What are mitochondria? https://www.medicalnewstoday.com/articles/320875

Wild Nutrition® Ltd. (2024, May 28). 8 Ways to support your mitochondria. https://www.wildnutrition.com/blogs/our-blog/8-ways-to-support-your-mitochondria

Pizzorno, J. (2014, April 1). Mitochondria—Fundamental to life and health. PubMed Central (PMC). https://www.ncbi.nlm.nih.gov/pmc/articles/PMC4684129/

Life Time. (2024, June 4). The care and feeding of your mitochondria. Experience Life. https://experiencelife.lifetime.life/article/the-care-and-feeding-of-your-mitochondria/